KANDI'S KICK-ASS GUIDE TO LIFE WITH PMDD

K. Torrence MSN, APRN, NP-C

Table of Contents

K. Torrence © 2024

"I think realizing that you're not alone, that you are standing with millions of your sisters around the world is vital." - *Malala Yousafzai*

My Breaking Point

I am sitting in a white plastic lawn chair on my

boyfriend's front porch. My head is spinning, and I feel

out of control. I look down and see my hands cut and

bleeding in my lap. The police officer says something

that snaps me back to attention. I look up at him. "Have

you thought of counseling, Miss?" I did not answer, just

K. Torrence © 2024

nodded, tears streaming down my face. I look over and

see my boyfriend standing on the other end of the porch

talking with the other police officer; he looks like he is

in pain, anguish even. "I don't want to press charges," I

hear him say. "I just want her to realize she needs some

help, something is wrong with her." "We understand,"

the police officer replies. "We recommend you stay

here, and for her to go back to her house for the

remainder of the night to let things cool down." "Yes,

sir," he replies. The second officer comes over to me.

"Miss, we recommend you return to your home for the

remainder of the evening to let things cool down. Your

boyfriend is concerned for your welfare and is not going

to press charges; however, we do strongly recommend

that you seek counseling." "Yes, sir," I reply. I sit there

in a daze wondering how the hell this all happened. The officer snaps me back to attention again. "Miss, do you need help to your vehicle?" "No, sir." I hurry to my feet and head toward my car. I look back, and my boyfriend is still talking with the police officer as I back out of the driveway. How the hell did this all happen? Will he ever forgive me? I think back. We were on the phone having a heated argument and he hung up on me. I remember feeling so furious I could not sit still. I was shaking all over. I tried calling him back, no answer. I called again, no answer. That motherfucker hung up on me! I became angrier and felt like I was just seething with rage. *I will show that fucking son of a bitch*, I thought. So, what happened next? I drove over to his house and shattered his doorway window out with a landscaping rock after he did not answer the door. Both of my hands were cut with shards of glass. I was so full of rage and adrenaline; I did not even realize I had been cut. "What the fuck is wrong with you!" he shouted. "You are fucking bleeding, look at your hands!" he shouted. "I almost fucking shot you!" he screamed again. "I called 911 because someone was breaking in, and I could have fucking shot you! What is wrong with you? You could fucking be dead right now!" he shouted. "This is not you. This is not the woman I fell in love with. Something is wrong!"

I pull into my driveway, turn off the engine, and close my eyes as everything replays in my head. I just sit there and cry. Something is wrong with me. I have never felt this out of control before in my life. I could have gone to jail, or worse, I could be fucking dead. He could

have shot me. I have never ever gotten into trouble with

law enforcement or been arrested before. I have never

been this angry or on edge before. I do not know what

came over me. I called the next morning and scheduled

an appointment with a therapist and a psychiatrist.

"Life is tough, my darling, but so are you."

- Stephanie Bennett-Henry

[CHAPTER 1] WHAT IS PMDD?

If you are reading this book, there is a good chance you already know what PMDD is. I, however, lived years of my life not knowing what PMDD is or that such a thing even existed. I knew that I occasionally had a rough menstrual cycle now and then, but most women do, right? Nothing could prepare me for the monthly monster that would soon creep in and destroy my life as I knew it. And destroy everything in my life it did.

K. Torrence © 2024

Relationships, friendships, jobs, and just life in general. PMDD is like the worst nightmare you could ever imagine coming to visit you regularly. Every. Single. Month. Does your life seem to be a huge dumpster fire living on an endless roller coaster that you cannot seem to escape? You may have PMDD. I want to dedicate this book to all the women and individuals who suffer from this gut-wrenching disorder. There is a way out. There is light at the end of the tunnel. Knowledge is power. This is my kick-ass guide to reclaiming your life and fighting that monthly battle with your nemesis, PMDD. You may not feel strong now, but you will be.

So, what exactly is PMDD? The American Psychiatric Association defines premenstrual dysphoric disorder (PMDD) as a severe form of PMS in which symptoms of anger, irritability, and internal tension are prominent.[1] It's a condition that causes severe emotional symptoms, such as extreme anger, anxiety, depression, and mood swings which occur the week of or two weeks before the menstrual period begins. My symptoms start with ovulation and continue to build until my period begins, sometimes even a few days after. Symptoms habitually turn ON and turn OFF each month. Anger and irritability are the most common among the behavioral symptoms of PMDD. Other behavioral symptoms include extreme sadness, hopelessness, sensitivity to rejection, anxiety/tension, and sometimes rage. PMDD symptoms are severe in nature and make it extremely difficult for the woman to function in everyday life. PMDD causes extensive personal suffering, occupational impairment, and disruption of interpersonal and family relationships.[20] These factors may combine, which can become life-threatening and increase the risk of suicide among affected individuals. PMDD is a strong risk factor for suicide, increasing the likelihood of suicide attempt and ideation by almost sevenfold and fourfold, respectively.[2]

What causes PMDD? The exact cause is unknown. Researchers suggest it is due to an ABNORMAL response to the normal cyclic hormone fluctuations that occur during each menstrual cycle. Circulating levels of ovarian hormones in people with PMDD have been found to fall in the standard range, suggesting that this disorder is not linked to a hormone imbalance, but rather to a heightened sensitivity in the brain.[3] Some studies suggest it is due to a sensitivity to estrogen, progesterone, and/or serotonin, as SSRIs have been proven effective in treating the symptoms of PMDD. Certain individuals may have increased risk factors making them more susceptible to developing the condition. Risk factors include a history of trauma or abuse, family history of PMS/PMDD, depression, or other mood disorders. Studies show menstruating women who smoke cigarettes are more likely to have PMDD symptoms, as well as individuals with seasonal affective disorder. Brain imaging in individuals with PMDD also reveal changes in gray matter and functioning compared to normal individuals. It is estimated that 3-8% of women in the reproductive age have PMDD, which causes a severe decrease in the quality of life and psychological problems.[5] I, personally, think this number is very inaccurate, as most individuals with PMDD go untreated and undiagnosed, especially in middle- to lower-class populations. Access to care remains an issue, although it is improving with the integration of telemedicine and online therapy, which is easily accessible at home. Even with more easily accessible care, there continue to be barriers to proper diagnosis. PMDD is under-recognized by health care providers, can be difficult to diagnose, and lies at the intersection of gynecology and psychiatry. Thus, patients can be misdiagnosed, or encounter challenges in seeking care.[16] Women are often desperate for help by the time they reach a physician with awareness of PMDD.[6] In addition, the knowledge and screening for

PMDD may still not be well known among healthcare providers. In the past three decades, the application of modern science and technology to investigate PMS and PMDD has lagged significantly behind that of other diseases.[7] The training for and familiarity with PMDD can vary widely among healthcare providers. Are they up to date with their continuing medical education? Do they have experience in the screening and management of PMDD? Some healthcare providers may not. Studies suggest mental health therapists, psychiatrists, and gynecologists all have the most skilled training and experience with PMDD management. I can tell you from personal experience that sometimes when it comes to our own or our family's health, we can be blinded. I am an urgent care provider. Yes, I had heard of PMDD way back in my medical training, but had not had any experience with diagnosis or management of PMDD due to the type of clinic I worked in. We treated mostly colds, flu, strep, sinus infections, minor lacerations, urinary tract infections—the list goes on with a variety of minor to moderate conditions. After I was diagnosed, it was like everything finally became clear to me, and I was not blind to the fact that my ship would have indeed been at the bottom of the ocean had I not sought professional help. And NO. You are NOT crazy. So many mental health conditions go undiagnosed and untreated due to many factors, including stigma and knowledge deficit. It can be exceedingly difficult to realize you may have an issue. Our brains can play tricks on us. How do we realize we may not be thinking normally or responding emotionally in a normal way if we do not understand what normal is or feels like? Research shows brain activity is DIFFERENT in individuals with PMDD versus a "normal" individual. This is a REAL, serious, and DISTRESSING disorder that can ruin lives if not diagnosed and treated.

PMDD snuck up on me. I had been on birth control pills since my teens. Birth control can be an effective option for treating PMDD. So, I was actually being treated for a condition I did not even realize I had. When did my symptoms show up? Mid-thirties, when I came off the birth control. There were lots of other stressors going on at that time in my life, including divorce and an incredibly stressful work environment, to which I attributed my symptoms. My symptoms continued to escalate until I reached my breaking point.

It can be so difficult to accept something is not right and

realize your mood, emotions, and behaviors can be

irrational. So, what does it FEEL like to have PMDD? It

HONESTLY depends on the day. Waking up with

PMDD is like flipping a fucking coin because you do

not know if it is going to be heads or tails. Good day or

bad day. You may wake up one morning feeling so

overcome with sadness and not understand why. And to

the EXTREME. You could be feeling okay one minute

and the next your boyfriend does some tiny little thing

that irritates you and you full on EXPLODE on him with

anger and rage. Over something stupid. It is like you

have no control whatsoever over your emotions and

mood. The closer I got to my period, the more I felt like

a ticking bomb just waiting to explode at any random moment. It is such an awful feeling. You are so anxious and full of adrenaline; it can be difficult to relax and be happy even when you do not have a reason to be upset. Another random day, you may wake up so tired and fatigued you cannot make it out of bed to go to work. You may sleep and stay in bed for hours or even days feeling depressed and hopeless. Then, once your period starts, you make a miraculous recovery and feel as if you are well and happier than you have ever been in your life. You are motivated and productive at work. You are more social and friendly and pleasant to be around. You are less argumentative and difficult to deal with. You honestly feel so good, you think you are well, and you will stay feeling this way. Not true. The predictable shift

WILL happen. This is why logging your symptoms can help. You can see a monthly pattern surrounding your period, which helps confirm your diagnosis and allows you to better manage your symptoms.

What is it like living with someone who has PMDD? Rough as fuck, my boyfriend would say. I literally broke up with him every two weeks over any minor inconvenience the first year we were together. I put him through hell. I really did. Being close to someone with PMDD can be just as tough as having the condition itself. They are suffering with you. If you have a significant other or someone that cares for you, I urge you to praise and thank them daily, and especially when you are well. Go above and beyond for that special person who suffers with you each month. I remember my boyfriend telling me that before I was diagnosed, he felt as if he were my personal punching bag. He felt like I took everything out on him and made it seem as if everything going on with me was his fault. This can be a difficult position to be in, and I am thankful each day he did not decide to throw in the towel. Counseling can be beneficial to you AND your partner, because they are going through this as well as you.

"Sometimes things fall apart, so that better things can fall together." - Marilyn Monroe

[CHAPTER 2] THE DANGER ZONE

The second half of every month is what my partner and I

refer to as "The Danger Zone." It can have many names.

The possibilities are endless! Some of the best names I

have read about include shark week, hell week, Mr.

Hyde's visit (referring to Dr. Jekyll/Mr. Hyde). This is

the second half of the menstrual cycle called the luteal

phase. This is when my symptoms turn ON and are the

most severe. During this time, my partner and I have

found it critical to be super aware of how I am feeling

and checking in with each other daily to help keep my

symptoms in check. Self-awareness is key. Since I have

been accurately diagnosed and treated, I have learned

more about myself and am more in-tune with my body

than I ever had been before. To be honest, I was

completely oblivious for a long time. You can have so

many symptoms with PMDD that you may have sought

treatment via many different providers, such as a

counselor, your primary care doctor, or even a

gynecologist. The correct diagnosis is so important,

because it allows you understand what is happening to

your mind and body every month. If we do not know or

understand what is happening, how can we do anything

about it? Unfortunately for me, I was oblivious to the fact that there was something wrong with me. It took over a year for me to connect the dots and realize it was connected to my menstrual cycle. I was in denial for a long time and thought I could deal with it and get well on my own. I am a very independent person, always have been. When you have work, kids, and are so busy with life in general, sometimes we can be blind to what is happening until the bomb drops and something happens that forces you to become aware and face the situation. Face the facts. Something is not right. What should you do? See your physician, gynecologist, or mental health provider. Only a licensed professional can diagnose you, as there are specific assessments that must be done to screen you for the condition. If you are reading this book, you most likely have already been diagnosed. What next? Discuss treatment options with your healthcare provider that best fit your needs. Consider your monthly cycle in comparison to the cyclic changes that occur in the ocean due to the moon's location and gravitational pull. Your hormones are constantly shifting and changing throughout each month as you progress through each phase of your cycle, just as the ocean is constantly moving and shifting. Even though we cannot see the moon's gravitational pull, we can see the effect it has on the ocean. The same is true with PMDD. We cannot visually see those hormones shifting each month, but we can feel and see the effects they have on our mind/body. I find so many things similar with standing in the ocean. The waves are constantly moving and shifting around you. You must

be present in the moment and aware of yourself and

surroundings. If you look away, you may be overtaken

by a large wave. If you stay aware, you will see that

wave coming, and you can prepare and swim right

through it.

"Girls should never be afraid to be smart."

- Emma Watson

[CHAPTER 3] ASS-KICKING TREATMENTS FOR PMDD

MEDICATIONS AND VITAMINS FOR PMDD

There are studies on prescription and non-prescription medication that have been proven to reduce the symptoms and severity of PMDD for many individuals. Among these are oral contraceptives, SSRIs, mood stabilizers, and certain vitamins. Oral contraceptives, or "birth control pills," help by stabilizing the monthly hormone shifts, which helps reduce symptoms and prevent ovulation. For patients over the age of 35, oral contraceptives are not a good option due to the increased risk of blood clots. SSRIs belong to a group of medications used to treat depression, anxiety, and other mental health conditions that multiple studies have proven effective for PMDD. Fluoxetine, also known as Prozac, is an SSRI that has shown rapid improvement in the symptoms of PMDD in as little as three days.[3] This is an interesting finding that is unique to PMDD. For patients with depression, it can take three to four weeks of treatment with fluoxetine to see improvements. This rapid onset of action is believed to be due to the serotonin sensitivity of those with PMDD.[3] Serotonin is a neurotransmitter or "messenger" naturally found in the brain involved in controlling mood and other functions.

Fluoxetine has definitely been a game changer for me. It

quickly helped turn my life around and improved my

day-to-day functioning. Some patients benefit from only

taking fluoxetine while in the luteal phase. I, however,

function the best taking fluoxetine daily throughout the

month with a slight dose increase while in my luteal

phase. I can function and deal with daily stressors while

feeling more stable throughout each monthly cycle.

Every person and how they respond to medication is

different. This is why it is so important to track your

symptoms and develop a plan of treatment with your

healthcare provider. What works for me may not work

for you. Everyone is different. The fluoxetine really

helped improve my PMDD, but there would be times

that I would still feel anxious and have difficulty

sleeping. Another add on medication my provider and I

have found to GREATLY improve all my symptoms has

been quetiapine. Quetiapine, or Seroquel, is an atypical

anti-psychotic medication used to treat many disorders

such as bipolar disorder, depression, and even

schizophrenia, because it helps stabilize mood and

promote sleep. I have to say I was a little skeptical at

first. I had found a few studies showing it to be

effective, but I was a little fearful of the "anti-psychotic"

drug class. My provider reassured me it would be worth

a try, and I have to say he was right! These two

medications have been my lifeline for controlling my

PMDD. Ovulation suppression is another option, with

the combined oral contraceptive pill (COCP) or GnRH

(gonadotropin-releasing hormone) agonists.[9] Leuprolide is a GnRH agonist that suppresses ovulation by inducing early menopause and may be used on a trial period before considering surgical removal of the ovaries.

There are also multiple vitamins that have been shown to be effective in improving PMDD symptoms. Vitamin B6 may help improve mood and wellbeing. I personally have found many benefits from taking a magnesium supplement as well. Magnesium is a mineral and a smooth muscle relaxant that helps improve mood and sleep. It is a regular in my daily regimen. Other supplements I have found to be beneficial include chasteberry and saffron. I found a recent study about how saffron is comparable to fluoxetine and just as effective in some patients. I immediately added this to my regimen and have found my symptoms even more

reduced. It also seems to lighten the flow of my periods,

which is an added positive! Given the recent social

media attention of the use of antihistamines for PMDD,

I would like to discuss that as well. I have not found any

studies on the efficacy of antihistamines for the

treatment of PMDD. Still, I can see how antihistamines

such as Hydroxyzine may help improve PMDD

symptoms due to their anti-anxiety benefits.

Surgical removal of the ovaries is another option

for treatment, which is only recommended as a last

resort in severe cases that have not responded well to

other treatment options. How does surgery help? It stops

ovulation and induces menopause by removing the

organs responsible for secreting female sex hormones.

Again, surgery should only be considered as a last resort

option due to surgical risk factors such as blood clots.

Inducing menopause early would mean hormone

replacement therapy to help manage menopausal

symptoms and prevent bone loss. Hormone replacement

therapy is also associated with increased risks of breast

cancers and blood clots.

NON-MEDICATION TREATMENT MEASURES

I cannot stress this enough—while taking your

medications as prescribed is particularly important, the

non-medication interventions are EQUALLY as

IMPORTANT. The following are things I have learned

through therapy, trial and error, books, and the research

K. Torrence © 2024

I have done to relieve stress and promote wellbeing.

- Self-awareness
- Sunlight
- Hydration and nutrition
- Avoid cigarette smoking
- Exercise
- Sleep
- Reduce sources of stress in your life.
- Aromatherapy.
- Acupuncture and massage therapy.
- Make time for hobbies you enjoy.
- Music therapy.
- Spend time with friends and family who make you happy.
- Enjoy your work.
- Counseling
- Reduce sources of stress in your life
- Make your home a place of peace and relaxation
- Consider an emotional support animal
- Candlelight
- Holiday survival guide—cannot stress enough how much this helped me!
- Forgiveness
- Boundaries
- The luteal phase

Self-Awareness

Self-awareness is defined as becoming aware of feelings in the moment—such as paying attention to physical sensations of emotional states—and is key to changing thoughts and behaviors.[24] Learning to practice self-awareness has been my most valuable tool. You must be able to recognize how you are feeling so that you are able to implement your self-care measures to help improve your mood and overall wellbeing. Check in with yourself daily and keep notes or a journal with the following questions. How is my mood today? Do I feel stressed, anxious, on edge? Do I feel more fatigued and tired than normal? Do I feel my heart racing? It is important to track your symptoms daily. PMDD is

PREDICTABLE. Stay on high alert when you are entering the luteal phase. If you are aware of how you are feeling, you can help improve your symptoms before they worsen—keep yourself in check, basically. Be sure to track your menstrual period. There are so many apps available that allow you to track and make notes of your symptoms, which makes it even easier to keep track of your cycle.

Sunlight

Given that light has strong, direct effects on mood, cognition, alertness, performance, and sleep, light can be considered a "drug" to treat many clinical conditions.[23] Individuals who suffer from seasonal affective disorder are at an increased risk for PMDD. While I have never been diagnosed with this, I can tell you that sunlight

helps me so much. I can see and feel a noticeable

difference in my mood and energy when I can be

outdoors in the sunlight. It feels so good to sit on my

porch drinking coffee with the morning sun shining on

my face. I have made this a daily habit to sit outside

each morning, weather permitting. Sunlight also

provides your body with essential vitamin D.

Hydration and nutrition

Adequate hydration and nutrition are important in

maintaining your health. It is recommended to follow a

healthy food model, in which fresh, unprocessed foods

predominate.[13] With PMDD, there are certain things that

can worsen your symptoms, such as excessive alcohol

intake, excessive carb and sugar intake, and excessive caffeine intake. Studies prove these factors can negatively affect your PMDD and worsen your symptoms. I have found it extremely helpful to avoid these things during my luteal phase.

Avoid cigarette smoking

Smoking is clearly associated with increased PMS/PMDD symptoms.[25] Tobacco affects the regulation of the sex hormones estrogen, progesterone, and androgens, which play a crucial role in the symptomology of PMDD.[25] If you smoke, quitting may greatly improve your symptoms and quality of life.

Exercise

Exercise is recommended by the American College of Obstetrics and Gynecology for reducing and managing PMDD symptoms, offering benefits like improved hormonal balance and psychological well-being.[15,26] Exercise stimulates our bodies to produce "feel good" hormones known as endorphins, which have been proven to improve mood and fight against stress, anxiety, and depression. It makes sense that staying active helps keep an increased level of these hormones circulating, which helps you feel better. I feel my best when I am active and am maintaining my workouts regularly. Aerobic exercise has been shown to be the most effective with improving PMDD symptoms. Although it can be challenging to get a workout in during my luteal phase, I try to not be super hard on myself and just go for a walk or short hike with my doggie. Anything that gets you outdoors and the blood pumping can be enough to help with your symptoms. So, if you are not feeling an intense 20–30-minute workout, don't be super hard on yourself! Getting any sort of physical activity while you are not feeling well is better than none. I have noticed I always feel improved afterward. Like most runners say, the first mile is the hardest! Do not give yourself time to think or talk yourself out of it, just get up and get moving. You will be glad you did!

Sleep

In the premenstrual phase, women with PMDD can experience insomnia, memory problems, difficulty maintaining focus, and fatigue.[27] Getting adequate sleep and maintaining a regular sleep routine is a must to help reduce and prevent exacerbation of your PMDD symptoms. When I have not gotten an appropriate amount of sleep, I notice a negative change in my mood and symptoms. I have found that I absolutely LOVE going to bed EARLY. Maintaining a regular bedtime routine can be highly effective. Set a time to put away all electronics, phones, and TV at least one hour prior to your bedtime. This will help you fall asleep faster, as your brain will be less stimulated and more ready for sleep. I have never been a morning person. But now, I can wake up and be ready to start my day a little easier by keeping my same early bedtime routine and allowing myself plenty of time for restful sleep. Magnesium and melatonin are also supplements that can help promote

sleep and relaxation.

Aromatherapy

Aromatherapy can be beneficial for management of such

symptoms as pain, nausea, vomiting, anxiety,

depression, stress, and insomnia.[28] I never knew what a

difference this would make in my life! Shower every

morning with your favorite fragrant soap/body wash and

take a relaxing bath every night before bed. Lavender

essential oil is very soothing for me. My therapist first

recommended this to me to help self-soothe when

feeling upset or on edge. Your favorite scent can help

relax you and bring you into the now. It can help

improve your mood and make you sleep better at night!

I love going to sleep with fresh lavender oil on my wrists or pillow.

Acupuncture and massage therapy

Acupuncture and acupressure may improve both physical and psychological symptoms.[22] I had never tried acupuncture before PMDD. It was an interesting experience for me, because I am a healthcare provider and am always curious about such things. Acupuncture is used in traditional Chinese medicine, which I have found remarkably interesting. Tiny needles are inserted to certain areas of the body which are believed to stimulate a healing response and possible release of endorphins. I've had friends ask, doesn't it hurt? For me, it did not. The acupuncture needles are very thin, tiny, just enough to elicit that healing response needed in the body. Acupuncture and massage are extremely relaxing for me and helped with low back pain as well.

Music therapy

Music therapy is another beneficial self-soothing strategy. There have been times I have felt completely overwhelmed and overstimulated while sitting in the noisy overcrowded airport. Music was my saving grace. Popping in my earbuds and listening to my favorite relaxing tunes helps me redirect my thoughts from what is overstimulating me and helps calm my senses.

Counseling

Counseling helped me learn ways to support and care for myself. It also taught me strategies that help reduce my symptoms when feeling on edge. It is amazing how so many little things you never thought of can help so much. I wish I would have sought counseling sooner. Before counseling, I relied on friends and family members. This is not a promising idea for the simple reason that they are not a licensed therapist with your best interests and mental health in mind. I feel like I suffered a great deal due to inappropriate advice and people pleasing. I was not good at setting boundaries. When you have PMDD, you can be so SUPER sensitive to rejection and other people's opinion of you. I suffered a lot due to this. Learning to put myself and my mental health needs first finally allowed me to be able to put

needed boundaries in place.

Emotional support animal

I have a miniature pinscher that I rescued from the local

animal shelter when she was six weeks old. She has

absolutely been my best friend and baby girl throughout

many challenging times in my life. People who have

never experienced trauma may not realize how having a

support animal really helps. For me, having her sit in my

lap wagging her little tail and giving me kisses helps

bring me to the present. When you are feeling anxious,

depressed, or on edge—unable to get circulating

thoughts and worries off your mind—she brings me to

the now. It is like I forget everything that is stressing me out. Having a support animal makes me feel loved

unconditionally and is more soothing to me than any

other thing. Whether you have had a dreadful day or are

in a horrible mood, they still love you and are happily

waiting to greet you when you arrive home.

Reduce extra sources of stress in your life

This is easier said than done. You may have many

sources of stress in your life you do not even realize you

have the control to reduce or eliminate. In the beginning,

I was horrible at setting and maintaining boundaries.

Over time, I toughened up when I realized how much

this protected my peace and stress levels. I also cut

many people out of my life. I do not even feel bad about

it. If certain people make your life worse and more

dramatic, you are not required to continue to allow them access to you. You are not required to give them an explanation. I did not. I felt like I did not owe anyone anything. I was doing what was necessary to survive and protect myself and improve my mental health. I also stopped using social media. This may not be for everyone, but it has changed my life for the better. This again greatly limited the access people had to me. No notifications. No bullshit. Just peace. I honestly do not even know that I would have a cell phone if it were not for my children. I always want to be accessible for them in case of emergency.

Make your home a place of peace and relaxation

K. Torrence © 2024

Surround yourself with décor, comfortable pillows, and any objects that make you feel happy in your space.

Keep it clean. I feel better when my house is clean, and I sleep better when my house is clean. Add candles! I discuss this in next section as ambiance helps promote relaxation. Make your space cozy, comfortable, with pics you love, and relaxing smells. Pamper yourself!

Candlelight

Candlelight has been proven to relax the body and mind. The flickering light creates a warm, calming ambiance. Not only candles can do this, even a campfire or hearth emits the same ambiance and warmth. Always be safe and abide by safety guidelines when burning candles or having a fire.

Make time for hobbies you enjoy

Make time for hobbies you enjoy! I love hiking and being outdoors in nature. I also love painting, music, and good books! Don't let PMDD keep you from the things you love! I also recommend carving out time in your schedule each week to spend time with friends/family.

Enjoy your work.

If you are not happy with your current job, it is easier than you might think to find one that suits you better. This is a big one that can help reduce your daily stress levels and improve your life in so many ways.

Holiday survival guide

When you have PMDD, the holiday season can be a huge trigger and source of stress for you. I dreaded being around certain family members to the point I wanted call in sick to the yearly family Christmas dinner. I don't enjoy being around people who make me feel uncomfortable or give off a bad vibe. I just don't. My therapist said pay attention to how you feel after you have spent time with someone. This is so true. If a particular person or family member makes you feel less than, limit the amount of time you spend with that person and realize their bad vibe has more to do with THEM and not YOU. Navigating the holiday season is all about setting and upholding your boundaries, which help keep your wellbeing and mental health intact.

K. Torrence © 2024

Setting boundaries can be difficult when you are overly

sensitive. Most people do NOT like boundaries, because

the boundaries do NOT benefit THEM. They only

benefit the person setting the boundaries. This is NOT

selfish at all. This is essential to protect your peace. If

you know you will be around your miserable cousin

Karen at Christmas who is the cunt of the century, limit

the amount of time you will spend there and uphold any

boundaries if she—or anyone—says something

untoward. A lot of people think family members will

always love you, support you, and have your best

interests in mind. This is NOT true. If you have a

wonderful, supportive, and mature family, that is great.

However, stressful, and non-ideal family situations and

conflicts have been some of the biggest sources of stress

in my life. Setting boundaries with my family has been the most difficult but most rewarding step I have taken toward peace and loving myself for who I am. Does my family know I have PMDD? Yes and no. It is a very personal thing. My parents, whom I am closest to, know. Opening up to other family members whom you may not be comfortable with may only give them an opportunity to voice their opinion, which you may not want to hear. I grew up in a very remote portion of the Southeastern U.S. Many of my family members have strict religious beliefs, which can cause bias and stigma toward some conditions and disorders. "Oh, it is just the devil making you that way." While I do admit there are times during my luteal phase I feel I need an exorcism, this is simply not true. In fact, I need routine medical care, medication, a strict daily routine, sometimes counseling, and support to treat and improve my symptoms each month. Living with PMDD is DIFFICULT! Do what you gotta do to take care of YOU! You cannot pour from an empty cup, and you definitely can't care for your children or family if you can't care for yourself.

Forgiveness

Forgiveness is also a HUGE part of healing and acceptance. With PMDD, you likely have and possibly will make mistakes. You may manage a situation with extreme emotion and hurt the people you care about. While having PMDD does not excuse harmful behavior, understanding the cause of it can help you learn from mistakes and handle situations better in the future.

Realizing that you can be extremely sensitive and

emotional at times, and sometimes irrational, is

particularly important. What can you do help fix a

problem? Apologize. A heartfelt apology goes a long

way. Taking accountability for your behavior and

apologizing can work wonders and show the people you

care about that you feel remorse and know your

behavior was not acceptable. A difficult realization for

me to accept was the fact some relationships may be

beyond repair. But that's okay. Learning to move

forward, accept the past, and do the best I can each day

to be better has improved my life greatly. Don't give up!

You have to forgive yourself, too, for your mistakes and

show yourself love and compassion. You did not ask to have PMDD.

Boundaries

If you don't set and maintain personal boundaries, I urge you to start today! Set and maintain boundaries with everyone and everything. It is YOUR responsibility to protect your peace, state of mind, and mental health. This alone can change your life. It is like putting on a shield of armor to protect yourself from the world and all the people in it.

The luteal phase

Monitor yourself closely during the luteal phase. Track your symptoms and how you are feeling daily. Staying on high alert can help you better prepare for and manage

your PMDD symptoms during your cycle's most severe

phase.

"Let go of who you think you're supposed to be;

embrace who you are."-Brené Brown

K. Torrence © 2024

[CHAPTER 4] SURVIVING THE PIT OF DESPAIR AND PMDD

For me, the pit of despair is the time in my life when I was most unwell. Undiagnosed, untreated, out of control, with my life falling to pieces around me. I suffered mentally and physically, and so did those around me. It was a struggle to meet my basic needs from day to day. There would be two- to three-day stretches in which I would not get out of bed except to use the bathroom, which wasn't very much since I was

not eating or hydrating. My lips were chapped and dry.

The fatigue was insane. It took every ounce of energy I

could muster to shower. I would have to let my hair air

dry because I did not have enough strength to hold the

hair dryer up for that long. There would be days I would

awaken in my bed feeling so hopeless, like there was no

point in continuing life feeling this way. It is like your

mind and body are stuck in a prison you cannot escape,

and you do not know how to help yourself, and you

can't seem to control your feelings or state of mind. I

felt like a failure in every way possible. I felt as if I had

let my kids and family down and there was no way it

could be mended. Every relationship around me

suffered, which made me feel even more alone and

hopeless. Your mind tricks you into believing there is no way out. Simply not true. I made the first step by seeking counseling. My therapist helped me 110%. I honestly thought I was going crazy. It felt so unbelievably good to talk to a professional who understood what I was going through and knew how to help me. She was the first step in getting the correct diagnosis and helping me learn strategies to improve my mental health and mood. If you are currently feeling like you are stuck, I urge you to seek treatment with a professional, and do not give up. Every little thing I went through has taught me so much about my mind/body and self-awareness. While going through the journey of life, we are not always taught how to care for our mind and body in healthy ways. Sometimes we get so busy with life we forget about these things until we are forced to deal with them. Take one small step each day. Caring for yourself requires a multifaceted approach. As discussed in this book, there are multiple interventions you can do to improve your symptoms each day. Make a note of things which are most beneficial to you and improve your mood. Practice those things regularly. Prepare each month for your luteal phase. Remember to track your cycle and symptoms. Each new day can be a new opportunity to love and care for yourself and feel BETTER. You can learn to navigate these difficult shifts each month. You can reclaim YOUR life and fight this battle one step at a time. And while I am still fighting this battle every single month, I have never felt STRONGER.

K. Torrence © 2024

Did you find this book helpful in some way? I would LOVE to hear about it! Please take a couple minutes to leave a review. Honest reviews help readers find the right book for their needs while also establishing the legitimacy of the book itself and the author. Help me bring the struggles of PMDD to the forefront! PMDD is REAL, and we deserve to be heard.

Afterword

Being able to write this book and turn my dream into a

reality has been fulfilling and healing in so many ways. I

want to thank my partner and children for all the love

and joy they bring to my life and for continuing to love

and support me daily. I love you all! I want to thank all

K. Torrence © 2024

of my readers for your support. You are not alone. I

wish you all the most love, support, and happiness.

References

1.American Psychiatric Association. *Diagnostic and Statistical Manual of Mental Disorders*. 5th ed. Washington, DC: American Psychiatric Association; 2013.

2.Prasad, D., Wollenhaupt-Aguiar, B., Kidd, K. N., de Azevedo Cardoso, T., & Frey, B. N. (2021). Suicidal Risk in Women with Premenstrual Syndrome and Premenstrual Dysphoric Disorder: A Systematic Review and Meta-Analysis. *Journal of Women's Health (2002)*, *30*(12):1693–1707. https://doi.org/10.1089/jwh.2021.0185

3.Stiernman, L., Dubol, M., Comasco, E., Sundström-Poromaa, I., Boraxbekk, C. J., Johansson, M., & Bixo, M. (2023). Emotion-induced brain activation across the menstrual cycle in individuals with premenstrual dysphoric disorder and associations to serum levels of progesterone-derived neurosteroids. *Translational Psychiatry*, *13*(1):124. https://doi.org/10.1038/s41398-023-02424-3

4.Sundström-Poromaa, I., & Comasco, E. (2023). New pharmacological approaches to the management of

Premenstrual Dysphoric Disorder. *CNS Drugs*, *37*(5): 371–379. https://doi.org/10.1007/s40263-023-01004-9

5.Gao, M., Qiao, M., An, L., Wang, G., Wang, J., Song, C., Wei, F., Yu, Y., Gong, T., & Gao, D. (2021). Brain reactivity to emotional stimuli in women with premenstrual dysphoric disorder and related personality characteristics. *Aging*, *13*(15):19529–19541. https://doi.org/10.18632/aging.203363

6.Cary, E. & Simpson, P. (2024). Premenstrual disorders and PMDD - a review. Best Pract Res Clin Endocrinol Metab, *38*(1):101858. doi: 10.1016/j.beem.2023.101858. Epub 2023 Dec 28. PMID: 38182436.

7.Long, J., Wang, Y., Liu, L., & Zhang, J. (2022). The prominent role of the temporal lobe in Premenstrual Syndrome and Premenstrual Dysphoric Disorder: Evidence from multimodal neuroimaging. *Frontiers in Psychiatry*, *13*, 954211. https://doi.org/10.3389/fpsyt.2022.954211

8.Studer, E., Nilsson, S., Westman, A., Pedersen, N. L., & Eriksson, E. (2023). Significance and interrelationship of the symptoms listed in the DSM criteria for premenstrual dysphoric disorder. *Psychiatric Research and Clinical Practice*, *5*(3):105–113. https://doi.org/10.1176/appi.prcp.20220007

9.Dunphy, L., Boyle, S., & Wood, F. (2023). The multifactorial aetiology and management of premenstrual dysphoric disorder with leuprorelin acetate. BMJ Case Rep, *16*(12): e258343. doi: 10.1136/bcr-2023-258343. PMID: 38160030; PMCID: PMC10759027.

10.Basso, J.C., McHale, A., Ende, V., Oberlin, D.J., & Suzuki, W.A. (2019). Brief, daily meditation enhances attention, memory, mood, and emotional regulation in non-experienced meditators. *Behav Brain Res,* 356:208-220. doi: 10.1016/j.bbr.2018.08.023. Epub 2018 Aug 25. PMID: 30153464.

11.Carlini, S. V., Lanza di Scalea, T., McNally, S. T., Lester, J., & Deligiannidis, K. M. (2022). Management of Premenstrual Dysphoric Disorder: A scoping review. *International Journal of Women's Health, 14*:1783–1801. https://doi.org/10.2147/IJWH.S297062

12.Goyal, A., Raza, F.A., Sulaiman, S.A., Shahzad, A., Aaqil, S.I., Iqbal, M., Javed, B., & Pokhrel, P. (2024). Saffron extract as an emerging novel therapeutic option in reproduction and sexual health: Recent advances and future prospectives. *Ann Med Surg* (Lond),*86*(5): 2856–2865. doi: 10.1097/MS9.0000000000002013. PMID: 38694315; PMCID: PMC11060205.

13.Siminiuc, R., & Țurcanu, D. (2023). Impact of nutritional diet therapy on premenstrual syndrome. Front

Nutr,*10*:1079417. doi: 10.3389/fnut.2023.1079417.
PMID: 36819682; PMCID: PMC9928757.

14.Sundström-Poromaa, I., & Comasco, E. (2023). New
pharmacological approaches to the management of
Premenstrual Dysphoric Disorder. *CNS Drugs*,
37(5):371–379. doi: 10.1007/s40263-023-01004-9. Epub
2023 May 12. PMID: 37171547; PMCID:
PMC10212816.

15.Management of Premenstrual Disorders: ACOG
Clinical Practice Guideline No. 7. Obstet Gynecol. 2023
Dec 1;142(6):1516–1533. doi:
10.1097/AOG.0000000000005426. PMID: 37973069.

16.Hantsoo, L., Sajid, H., Murphy, L., Buchert, B.,
Barone, J., Raja, S., & Eisenlohr-Moul, T. (2022).
Patient experiences of health care providers in
Premenstrual Dysphoric Disorder: Examining the role of
provider specialty. *J Womens Health* (Larchmt),
31(1):100–109. doi: 10.1089/jwh.2020.8797. Epub 2021
Apr 1. PMID: 33978482; PMCID: PMC8785767.

17.Jackson, C., Pearson, B., Girdler, S., Johnson, J.,
Hamer, R.M., Killenberg, S., & Meltzer-Brody, S.
(2015). Double-blind, placebo-controlled pilot study of
adjunctive quetiapine SR in the treatment of
PMS/PMDD. Human Psychopharmacology. *30*(6):425–
34. doi: 10.1002/hup.2494. Epub 2015 Jul 19. PMID:
26193781.

18. Dilbaz, B., Aksan, A. (2021). Premenstrual syndrome, a common but underrated entity: Review of the clinical literature. J Turk Ger Gynecol Assoc. *22*(2):139–148. doi: 10.4274/jtgga.galenos.2021.2020.0133. Epub 2021 Mar 5. PMID: 33663193; PMCID: PMC8187976.

19. Kaltsouni, E., Fisher, P.M., Dubol, M., Hustad, S., Lanzenberger, R., Frokjaer, V.G., Wikström, J., Comasco, E., & Sundström-Poromaa, I. (2021). Brain reactivity during aggressive response in women with Premenstrual Dysphoric Disorder treated with a selective progesterone receptor modulator. *Neuropsychopharmacology, 46*(8):1460–1467. doi: 10.1038/s41386-021-01010-9. Epub 2021 Apr 29. PMID: 33927343; PMCID: PMC8209206.

20. Parry, B.L., Meliska, C.J., Martinez, L.F., Lopez, A.M., Sorenson, D.L., Dawes, S.E., Elliott, J.A., & Hauger, R.L. (2023). A 1-week sleep and light intervention improves mood in Premenstrual Dysphoric Disorder in association with shifting melatonin offset time earlier. *Arch Womens Ment Health, 26*(1):29–37. doi: 10.1007/s00737-022-01283-z. Epub 2022 Dec 15. PMID: 36520251; PMCID: PMC9908689.

21. Tiranini, L., & Nappi, R. E. (2022). Recent advances in understanding/management of premenstrual dysphoric disorder/premenstrual syndrome. *Faculty Reviews, 11*;11. https://doi.org/10.12703/r/11-11

22. Armour, M., Ee, C.C., Hao, J., Wilson, T.M., Yao, S.S., & Smith, C.A. (2018). Acupuncture and acupressure for premenstrual syndrome. *Cochrane Database Syst Rev, 8*(8):CD005290. doi: 10.1002/14651858.CD005290.pub2. PMID: 30105749; PMCID: PMC6513602.

23. Wirz-Justice, A., Skene, D.J., & Münch. M. (2021). The relevance of daylight for humans. Biochem Pharmacol,*191*:114304. doi: 10.1016/j.bcp.2020.114304. Epub 2020 Oct 28. PMID: 33129807.

24. Iovino, E.A., Koslouski, J.B., & Chafouleas, S.M. (2021). Teaching simple strategies to foster emotional well-being. Front Psychol, *12*:772260. doi: 10.3389/fpsyg.2021.772260. PMID: 34858296; PMCID: PMC8631539.

25. Fernández, M.D.M., Montes-Martínez, A., Piñeiro-Lamas, M., Regueira-Méndez, C., & Takkouche, B. (2019). Tobacco consumption and premenstrual syndrome: A case-control study. PLoS One, *14*(6): e0218794. doi: 10.1371/journal.pone.0218794. PMID: 31226148; PMCID: PMC6588233.

26. Liguori, F., Saraiello, E., & Calella, P. (2023). Premenstrual Syndrome and Premenstrual Dysphoric Disorder's impact on quality of life, and the role of physical activity. *Medicina* (Kaunas), 59(11):2044. doi:

10.3390/medicina59112044. PMID: 38004093; PMCID:
PMC10673441.

27. Lin, P.C., Ko, C.H., Lin, Y.J., & Yen, J.Y. (2021).
Insomnia, inattention and fatigue symptoms of women
with Premenstrual Dysphoric Disorder. *Int J Environ
Res Public Health, 18*(12):6192. doi:
10.3390/ijerph18126192. PMID: 34201084; PMCID:
PMC8230179.

28. Farrar, A.J., & Farrar, F.C. (2020). Clinical
Aromatherapy. *Nurs Clin North Am, 55*(4):489–504.
doi: 10.1016/j.cnur.2020.06.015. Epub 2020 Sep 28.
PMID: 33131627; PMCID: PMC7520654.